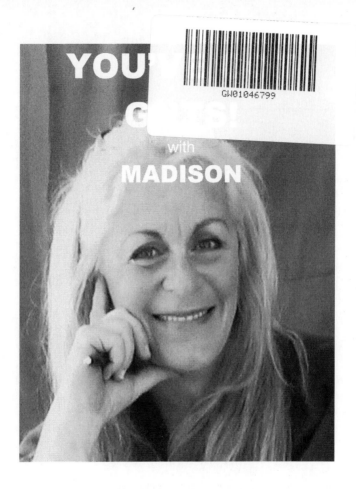

YOU...
G...
with
MADISON

The Western diet and an increasingly stressful lifestyle
can play havoc with our guts and IBS and stress related
digestive problems are on the increase.
Madison has prepared a short and simple commonsense
guide to a healthier digestive system.
Based on reviewing your diet, lifestyle and some great
energy medicine tips, it is an invaluable tool in your
quest for well being.

All paper used in the printing of this book has been made from wood grown in managed, sustainable forests.

ISBN: 978-1-78003-813-1

Essential Book Series

Printed and published in the UK
Author Essentials
4 The Courtyard
South Street
Falmer
BN1 9PQ

A catalogue record of this book is available from the British Library

Cover design © Author Essentials
info@authoressentials.com

The author can accept no responsibility for any accident, health problem or injury as a result of using the information in this book. It is not a substitute for consulting your doctor.
The material is intended for informational purposes, it is not prescriptive.
If are under medical supervision, please check with your healthcare practitioner before implementing any of the suggestions in this book.

CONTENTS

Introduction

This little book is going to take a look at a number of digestive problems, but perhaps top of the list of tummy 'grumbles' is IBS.

Irritable Bowel Syndrome is also known as Spastic Colon and is one of the most common conditions in contemporary Western society[1]. The NHS quote that 20% of people in the UK develop IBS at some stage in their life. Its increase may be attributable to two key factors:

a]   Our change in diet to more processed and chemical rich foods

b]   That old chestnut – stress. So many of us are like swans on water, on the surface we may appear calm, graceful and in control, yet underneath we are paddling around like crazy, trying to keep afloat.

IBS is a problem with the *function* of the intestine, rather than an abnormality of the organ itself, so the gut will appear normal if viewed, thus making it hard to diagnose accurately.

IBS is not life threatening but can be a source of great discomfort and inconvenience. Intensity of the symptoms can vary and even clear completely, so there is hope; and there is certainly a lot you can do for yourself.

---

[1] As is Candida, see Coping with Candida [Essential Books series]

If you have any concern at all, please talk to your doctor. A simple blood test can rule out conditions such as ulcers, colitis, celiac disease, anaemia or an infection; symptoms of which can be confused with IBS. Certainly, passing blood is _not_ a symptom of IBS and you should consult your doctor immediately. NICE identify 3 key symptoms by ABC – do you have:

Abdominal pain or discomfort?

Bloating?

Change in bowel habits?

There is no clear explanation of what exactly causes IBS but an awful lot of sufferers can relate the start of symptoms to an emotional upset or a particularly stressful episode in their life. What you eat and drink definitely affects the gut. Often symptoms can worsen after a course of antibiotics which will alter the balance and ratio of good/bad bacteria in the gut.

So, if you don't want your 'irritable' bowel to turn 'vindictive' furious and nasty' – take time to look after and calm it down.

I will talk briefly in the book about Celiac disease, food poisoning [gastro enteritis] and Crohn's but broadly speaking any of these will benefit from the techniques and information contained in this small book.

I will write separately about Liver and Gallbladder as although part of digestion their roles are some wide spread that I felt they deserved their own space.

What I would suggest is that you read through with an open mind and be discerning; if something 'sounds' right to you, try it and objectively assess if you feel better. You will probably feel a prickle of interest that draws you to what you need.

You have guts and I hope you find this book helps you take care of them.

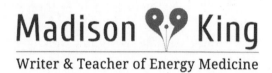

Writer & Teacher of Energy Medicine

What can go wrong?

One of the symptoms of a digestive problem is bad breath.

Check yours now.

IRRITABLE BOWEL SYNDROME [IBS][2]

Okay, so how will you recognise IBS?

Well first of all there may be bloating and perhaps wind. This can also be a symptom of sensitivity to wheat. If you exclude what for a while and the symptoms persist then you can suspect IBS.

There may also discomfort, or even pain or spasm in the abdominal area. This can come and go and can often ease when you go to the loo or pass wind.

You experience diarrhoea and equally constipation. Your bowels have lost their balance and will swing between these two extremes. There may well be an early morning urgent 'rush'.

Other hints will include:

- Feeling sick
- Headaches
- Belching
- Loss of appetite
- Tiredness
- Backache
- Heartburn

---

[2] *Further help and advice*
The IBS Network Tel: 0872 300 4537
Web: www.theibsnetwork.org

This is not a bowel that has got a bit of a 'paddy on', as they say on the Isle of Wight;[3] it is an actual medical condition and needs to be taken seriously.

CROHN'S INFLAMMATORY BOWEL DISEASE

Crohn's is less common, affecting about 1 in every 1200 people. We still do not know what causes it. It can strike anywhere between the mouth and the rectum – the entire digestive tract. It will start with inflammation, progressing to ulcers and scarring of parts of the intestinal wall.

The symptoms of Crohn's are more aggressive than IBS: pain, urgent diarrhoea, loss of weight and certainly tiredness. You may also suffer problems with inflamed joints and possibly skin [a lot of digestive problems can be reflected in the condition of your skin].

As a matter of interest, it is named after Dr Burril Crohn, who was part of the team who discovered the condition in 1932.

DIVERTICULITIS

Is more common, 50% of over 60's. It occurs in the large intestine and develops from diverticulosis [the formation of pouches on the colon. The 'itis' gives us a clue to what it is: an inflammation of one, or more, of those pouches [called diverticula] that can become infected by small pieces of food, for example

---

[3] *With immense respect to the IOW – my birthplace*

sweet corn or undigested meat morsels, trapped in them.

Symptoms include pain and tenderness, often in the lower left-hand side of the abdomen. Again diarrhoea or constipation may be present and possibly fever. If infection is involved then nausea, vomiting and cramping may also occur.

We still don't know exactly what causes this condition. Processed foods and not enough fibre can definitely contribute to the problem and maybe even cause it by causing constipation that can increase the pressure on the large intestine causing the pouches to form.

CELIAC DISEASE [GLUTEN INTOLERANCE]

For Celiac Disease we move to the small intestine, where damage is caused by a reaction to eating gluten [wheat, barley, rye and the jury is out on oats]. The reaction can damage the villi in the lining of the small intestine and prevent optimum absorption of nutrients. Effectively, whatever the sufferer eats they will eventually become malnourished, resulting in symptoms such as fatigue, diarrhea, weight loss and a general lack of well-being. A predisposition to Celiac can be inherited. It is relatively common as 1 in 133 people can suffer from it.

If you suspect you have Celiac, there is a really practical and informative site: www.celiac.com – food lists and recipes are available. To give you a feel of what you can and can't eat:

Foods that are allowed include: beans, seeds and nuts [unprocessed], eggs, fresh grilled meats, fish and poultry, fruit and vegetables. Moderate dairy [check labels]. Buckwheat, corn, flaxseed, Quinoa, Rice and the myriad gluten-free products that are available today.

You need to avoid: all food and drink containing: barley, malt, rye and o course, wheat, Bulgur and Spelt. Beer, bread, cakes, pies, cereals, croutons, sweets, pastas, salad dressings, sauces, soy sauce and crisps.

FOOD POISONING – GASTROENTERITIS

We've all picked up a little 'stomach bug' at some time in our life and know the misery of diarrhoea, vomiting and abdominal cramping and pain. If prolonged, dehydration can occur.

This is another 'itis' – inflammation this time that involves the stomach and small and large intestine. It can be viral or bacterial.

HEARTBURN

Very unpleasant and very common – up to 40% of people will experience this year. Heartburn occurs when acid from the stomach flows back up into the oesophagus and irritates the sensitive lining. There is a valve at the top of the stomach that should prevent this, however it can malfunction. It is also called reflux, oesophagitis or indigestion.

You may experience: burning pain behind the breastbone that can travel up the neck. Acid taste in the back of the throat or burping.

ULCERS

Stomach [gastric] ulcers are basically open sores that can develop on the lining of the stomach. They can also form on the duodenum [just beyond the stomach] and are known as duodenal ulcers. Both of these are sometimes called peptic ulcers.

They can be caused by bacteria, or drugs such as ibuprofen or aspirin and certainly consistent stress can make you vulnerable. Smoking can also irritate the lining. Ulcers are common in the West where it is estimated that 10% of the population may develop a stomach ulcer.

Common symptoms include a burning pain in the centre of the abdomen.

THE ROLE OF STRESS AND ANXIETY

Any one of the above digestive problems is exacerbated, or even caused, by stress, worry and anxiety. So it makes sense that if you want to feel better, you need to look at these aspects of your life before doing anything else. To be as free as reasonably possible from this turbulent triad unpins rather than undermines digestive health.

Whether we like it or not, stress is part of our life and, in my opinion, is part of the cause of almost everything that can go wrong with us, certainly too much stress inhibits our body's natural ability to balance and heal itself. Not all stress is damaging, we need a certain amount of stress to get us out of get out of bed in the morning and approach our day with at least a semblance of zesty vigour and enthusiasm.

If we rummage into the semantics; it is not so much the stress itself as our individual response to the 'stressor; how we react is what *actually* causes the damage, or as so many people call it; the 'di-stress'.

I suppose it is the same as with everything in life – moderation. A little stress is a positive thing – too much [and it is different for everyone] can undermine your core health.

The emotional, educational, financial, social, family and work aspects of our lives can all trigger anxiety and an inappropriate stress response. What is stressful for one person is a doddle for another. We each need to recognise what stresses us as individuals.

Our negative stress responses are very real, it is not just a case of being 'weak willed' or it all being 'in the mind'. It can impact physically on the body, especially along the digestive tract.

We have all experienced that tight knotting in our stomachs before we go for an interview, sit an exam, drive in busy traffic, the reality of budgeting when times are tight, queuing while in a rush. Or in my case, right now, the realisation of a deadline looming VERY soon!

Stress is a daily reality

Harness your response

Don't allow it be a daily disaster

Don't be an ostrich and fall into the trap of negative stress management: thinking you are a failure because you are stressed, therefore denying the problem: drinking too much; taking drugs;

overeating; over working; smoking or becoming an angry grump. None of these are an effective long term solution. In fact most aren't even a short term one.

Instead, look at positive stress management: meditation, relaxation, sport, and reading. Kindle playtime, even watching some light-hearted television or movies can help you step off the daily stress merry-go-round. Be careful what you watch though, I can remember reading about some research among students that when they were exposed to an uplifting programme their bodies reacted in a far healthier way than when they were exposed to an emotional documentary about war camps. Common sense really.

If you have a chance, read Masaru Emoto's book *The Hidden Messages in Water*. It introduces the work of this renowned Japanese scientist, who has discovered that molecules of water are affected by our thoughts, words and feelings and of course, what we expose ourselves to. Since we are composed mostly of water, it makes sense to expose ourselves only to positive, uplifting circumstances that make us smile and create a peaceful, nurturing environment in which to live, work and play.

I know, I know: you're thinking this is a little Pollyanna to say the least and certainly very difficult to achieve in our modern society; but we can try; at the very least we can eliminate some of the obvious negativity in our lives.

So next time someone cuts you up in traffic or some idiot queue jumps when you are in a hurry, or, my personal favourite: on a plane when the person next to you sneezes, snorts and coughs their germs all over you, without even the courtesy of a tissue to block almost certain contamination of all around him/her: *don't* dive head first into an aggressive response, don't 'tutt' yourself into stress, don't let rage rule you. Instead, take a breath, smile and have a peaceful 'keyword' that makes you smile.

KEYWORD formation. I have four I use regularly, partnered with a couple of seconds of deep breathing; they can stop me having an *inappropriate* stress response, such as screaming like a fishwife, or pursing my lips and involuntarily tightening my muscles. I say inappropriate because of course one can feel annoyed, irritated or angry – the secret is to let that emotion pass through your body quickly and freely, without getting stuck and causing self-harm. So I don't scream obscenities, my lips un-purse pretty quickly and my muscles relax. So what are my words?

1. Love
2. Peace
3. Let it go [and smile, even if you don't mean it]
4. And the third is not really a word, I imagine Eric Idle singing: *"Always look on the bright side of Life"*

Music can be incredibly uplifting and change the mood of anyone. If I am ever teaching something that is a little 'heavy' or I feel the energy of the class is becoming negative for any reason, I will often use music to lift the mood: Age of Aquarius, Que Sera Sera [Doris Day] or Wonderful World [Louis

Armstrong] – whatever appeals and gets people smiling.

Your personal keyword/s and music [play it in the car] are useful and free tools that can bring you back from the edge of a negative stress response. Put this book down right now and think of a word that may work for you: meadow, kitten, snowflake, and sandy beach – what word sparks an association with something that makes you feel really good?

What else could you do to help yourself?

- Go for a walk
- Curl up on the sofa with a good book
- Have a massage, facial or treatment of your choice
- Have a coffee with a friend that makes you laugh
- Sing, dance or both in front of the mirror – hairbrush microphone optional
- Take a scented bath – and talk gently to yourself, talk as if you were talking to a precious friend or child – be kind. Very few things are truly worth getting stressed about – talk yourself round to a different perspective

Bad things happen though and if all else fails, go through the stress and try and find the lesson in it because sometimes that is the secret key to release: understanding the message that a stressful person, situation brings you – sometimes they are only the messengers; and once you get the message the messenger goes away.

*An occasional sprinkle of manure on our gardens
can make the roses grow and glow!*

So these are commonsense things you can do for
yourself – not necessarily easy if you have created
bad stress response habits over the years; but
certainly something you can work with to loosen the
grip of those habits.

There are some great books out there on stress
busting. However, let me share with you now a few
of my personal favourite techniques that have their
roots in energy medicine. Try each one and see
which feels the most powerful for you; and then
simply use it.

They are:

- *Teddy Boy Sweep and Hook up*
- *Head Holding*
- *Cleopatra hold*
- *Empty out, zip and sew up* [4]
- *Letting go on a breath*

Teddy Boy Sweep

If ever I announce this
technique when I am
teaching in the US, I get
vacant stares from the
students; they imagine I am
talking about teddy bears or
Dick Van Dyke in *Mary
Poppins!* Not at all, I am of

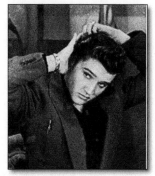

---

[4] Based on Donna Eden's Expelling the Venom exercise
featured in her book Energy Medicine

the age that remembers vividly the 'teddy boys', Elvis and James Dean. Imagine those boys combing their hair, up over their ears, sleeking it down at the sides and down behind their ears.

It is that motion that you imitate. Deceptively simple and very effective, this technique simply traces part of the Triple Warmer meridian [channel of energy] *backwards.*

These pathways of energy throughout the body are one-way streets and if you trace the energy *backwards* along the street, if you go in the 'wrong' direction, it has the effect of taking out excess energy, instantly sedating and calming the energy and in this case can instantly take the edge of any stress reaction. You will immediately feel calmer and more able to cope and your stress response will not be so damaging to your body.

As with all good techniques this one is easy to do, in fact many of us automatically run our hands through our hair, often blowing out at the same time. It is an instinctive human reaction to anxiety and stress. Here's how you do it:

- Place the palms of your hands over your temples, in front of your ears.

- Take a moment or two to tune into your 'energy', make a connection between the palms of your hands and what lies underneath them. Moving energy is something anyone can do: think of your hands as little electromagnetic pads and when you move them slowly, with focus and intention, over the body, the energy follows. Even a child [in fact children are really good at this] can easily move energy around a body.

- Take a deep breath and smile – I'm not being flippant here, but smiling encourages the release of endorphins in the body, so your body associates the Teddy Boy Sweep with something good – increasing your body's receptiveness to the technique and therefore its efficiency.

- Slide the palms up over and behind the ears, down the neck to the shoulders. Breathing out as you move down.

- Pause on the shoulders: your fingers will be over the top and back of the shoulders and the heels of each hand will be resting just above the collar bones. Remember to smile and you might like to close your eyes, which will help you 'sense' the energy.

- Take another deep breath and apply slightly more pressure, pull your hands off the body – to the front.

- Shake your hands off and repeat as many times as necessary until you feel calmer.

By the way, in the US, they have a great name for the haircut:
> *D.A. [duck's bottom].*

An optional ending to Teddy Boy Sweep, or a technique that can stand on its own is:

HOOK UP
Hyperlink to harmony

'Discombobulated'
... I simply love the sound of this word although I have my doubts as to its 'official' existence, just the sound of it manages to describe how we can all feel occasionally: Uncoordinated in both body and mind; a bit 'off'; a little 'spaced out'; stuck; not fully in the flow of life and unable to cope with the challenges life sets us.

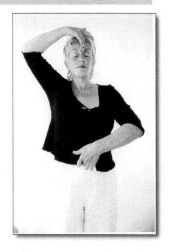

This simple technique is a hyperlink to harmony and balance. It connects [hooks up] two important channels of energies: Governing and Central. It brings clarity of thought and purpose; strengthens the auric field and bridges the energies between the head and the body. You will feel more connected, co‐ordinated, grounded and able to cope. It is particularly good to do after any 'stress technique', to help integrate the changes.

- Place the middle finger of one hand on your forehead between the eyebrows, over the 3rd Eye

- Place the middle finger of the other hand in your navel

- With a slight pull of the skin upward on both points, close your eyes, take a deep breath and relax. [Breathe in through the nose and out through the mouth] – smile, I know you might feel silly doing this but it does enhance effectiveness

- Stay in this position for about twenty seconds [or a few minutes, whatever feels right to you]

What are you actually doing? You are hooking up two key pathways of energy and making them stronger. By strengthening the *Governing Channel* that runs up the back, you affect the spine, not only in a physical sense but also in an emotional way – literally giving you the 'backbone' to face and resolve problems and move forward in your life. So much stress is caused by feeling helpless.

By strengthening the *Central Channel* that runs up the front of the torso you will be less vulnerable to absorbing other peoples' negative energies. An overdose of these can cause not only stress but also exhaustion and even depression.

It is a powerful tool for quickly cantering yourself and has immediate neurological consequences. It has been reported to be helpful to a person starting to seizure.

Put the book down and try it right now and see if you feel less discombobulated!

HEAD HOLDING

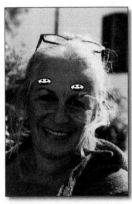

You could call this the '*Oh My God*' points as they are situated exactly where you would place your hand on your forehead when stressed. Halfway between your eyebrow and hairline in line with your eyes when they are looking straight ahead, these two points are your new best friends. Hold them with fingertips until you feel a pulse. This signals that the blood is moving from the back to the forebrain.

Excellent when problems seem insurmountable; when you are so deeply caught up in grief or concern. Hold the back of your skull for extra reassurance or if the stress overlaps into fear.

Cleopatra Hold

I believe we all do this without thinking, look at this photo of me, I think a bit of unintentional self-treatment was going on that day.

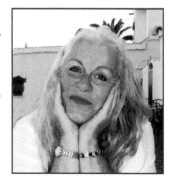

Rest your chin on the heels of your hands with the fingertips placed in a line running from edge of eye to ear – rather like Elizabeth Taylor's make up in Cleopatra.

Sit there for 30 seconds, smile and count your blessings – literally feel an attitude of gratitude.

What's happening? You are balancing the neurovascular points associated with Stomach [on the jaw line] and on the Cleopatra line you are affecting: Governing, Triple Warmer and Kidney.

What does that do? It reduces stress, anxiety and fear and increases courage and your ability to process problems.

If you are a therapist, hands will be reversed. Simply hold for a few minutes and you will begin to feel pulses while your client will be snoring.

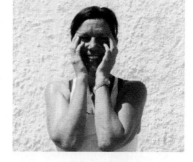

EMPTY OUT, ZIP AND SEW UP
disconnecting the 'thug' within

How many of us walk around priding ourselves on feeling, 'enlightened', civilised and in control? Not for us the explosive rage, angry outbursts, temper tantrums, irritated indignation, stress overwhelm or fits of frustration. Oh no, we have moved beyond all of that – or have we?

The other day I witnessed cruelty to a dog [I am not going into details or my bile will start rising again]. Suffice to say, in a nano second, I totally lost my temper at a cruel and ignorant 'owner'. It alarmed me to be reminded that I still have a huge potential for anger, my fuse may be extremely long, but once lit, it can flare up instantly and blind me to all reason. Everything I have learnt over the past couple of decades goes out the window as a cascade of wrath washes through me and I connect to the wild thug, rather than wise woman, inside.

Anger is natural; there is nothing wrong in feeling the full force of this emotion. It does not make you a bad person. However, what is bad for you is when this anger gets stuck inside and you are unable to let it pass through, out and on; it begins to dig roots and fester, causing *stress* within the body. So whether you are furious with the guy that has just cut you up at the traffic lights, or seething at yourself for not saying 'no' and therefore allowing yourself to be put into a stressful situation: it is wise to face your anger, feel it and let it go – life really is too short, will you remember that guy in 5 years time? Will the world end if you say 'no'?

The Chinese believe anger to be associated with Wood Element[5]. This Element also governs two key organs: the Liver [associated with *inwardly* directed anger, impatience and frustration] and the Gallbladder [associated with *outwardly* directed and 'harboured' anger, bottled up emotions, irritability, resentment and aggression]. Both these organs are crucial in your digestion.

For now, let's look at a way of expelling any stale residue of stressful emotions: anger, frustration, negativity, toxic thoughts and perhaps any

---

[5] Traditional Chinese Medicine and philosophy is based upon the 5 Elements: Water, Wood, Fire, Earth and Metal.

energetic 'gunk' you may have picked up from others or your environment.

Place hands over your head, arms straight, fists clenched, wrists crossed.

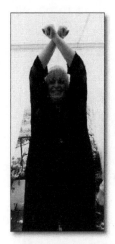

Breathing out, bring hands down quickly and with force, uncrossing and taking them out to the side of the thighs with fingers now outstretched, not clenched.

While doing this, imagine a line

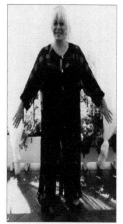

that runs down the centre of the body, from mouth to the genital area. Imagine this line opening up, becoming 'unzipped' and any anger, rage, irritation, or negative energetic 'gunk' that has been lurking inside finally spilling out into the earth.

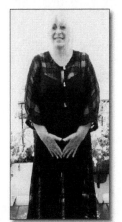

At the same time breathe out with a hissing sound and imagine all those angry toxic emotions, energies and thoughts spilling out on your breath.

Repeat 3 times

You are now 'open' and it is important to zip up that Central Meridian so that toxic energies that may be around you can no

22

longer enter and cause disruption. This zip up boosts confidence and positivity and clears your thoughts.

Simply place your hand at the bottom of the meridian [between your legs]. Take a deep in-breath and simultaneously move your hand up the centre

of the body to your lower lip and 'lock it' by lightly tweaking the sides of your mouth.

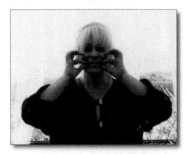

As you do this, think of calmness, forgiveness and tranquillity being zipped up inside

Do this 3 times and end by 'sewing up' i.e. tracing a horizontal Figure of 8 up the centre line, rather like an old fashioned Victorian corset.

This will give you a wonderful protection against external energies entering your body; against some of the stresses of life triggering unnecessary anger. It does not stifle you; you can still give out care, warmth, attention and love.

So next time the stress of a toxic temper, the Victor Meldrew in each of us, threatens to emerge, do a quick empty out and zip/sew up.

LETTING GO ON A BREATH

This exercise stimulates the Neurolymphatic points relating to the Lung and Large Intestine letting go] and draws on the power of visualisation to release negative elements [and people] from your life enabling you to let go of stress and move on.

- Firmly massage down the breastbone −about 5 seconds
- Move fingers to either side of the bone and massage firmly upwards − about 5 seconds
- Repeat 3 times − your are massaging points related to the Lung

- Firmly massage down the outside of the thigh [where the trouser seam sits], in a straight line from top of thigh to just above the knee. You can do both thighs at the same time.
- Repeat 3 times − you are massaging points related to the Large Intestine

- Take a deep breath and relax
- Bring to mind the person, situation, negative element or emotion you want to release from your life
- Exhale and imagine you are blowing him/her/it out of your inner depths
- Repeat 3 times

- Now for the extra piece of magic…

- Cup hands together in front of chest/neck area and imagine the person, situation, or representation of the emotion sitting there in your hands − about the size of a chess piece
- Inhale deeply and as you very slowly exhale, visualise him/her/it being blown away, scattering into the wind and disappearing into the distant horizon.[6] At the same time thinking *"xyz leave*

---

[6] Needless to say, this is not an exercise to be done in front of your mirror!

my life, in love and in the most divine way –
GOODBYE, go in peace"

- Take a couple of deep breaths and smile – try ending with the exercise empty out and zip up [above]

I was shown the basis of this technique on the Island of Gozo[7], on the cliffs overlooking the sea – a perfect location to let go of negativity, send it back to the earth [her ability to take the negative and transform it]or the ocean/water [cleansing/new beginnings].

So this gives you a few basic tools to combat the effect of stress on your digestion, in fact on all your systems. Try each one and see which delivers results for you. [8]

Importance of diet in general

Hippocrates the father of Western Medicine said that

"our food should be our medicine"

Develop your own personal digestive medicine.

What your put into your digestive tract is obviously going to have a tremendous impact on it, so it is crucial that you take time to honestly evaluate your diet. Let go of focussing only on what makes you fat

---

[7] Thank you Dr Sara for sharing this all those years ago, I always think of you with a smile when I do it.

[8] For a wider selection of energy exercises try my little book: *Everyday Energy* or Donna Eden's *Energy Medicine.*

and start paying attention to what makes your body feel good and what doesn't, through observation, learn what foods trigger a bad digestive response in you.

There are many lists, rules and common sense guidelines, but a really reliable way of 'fine tuning' your diet is to learn to energy test yourself and only eat foods that test strong for you. If you are not confident with self testing [and many people are doubtful of their abilities] then simply go the elimination of the obvious + observation route. Both are well worth the effort.

New research is published every month often with conflicting findings – so what do you believe? Believe how you _feel_, trust your instinct; objectively evaluate results of any changes you make – that is the only effective way of devising a diet that makes you feel great!

The keywords when formulating your personal eating plan are:

Commonsense/moderation/rotation/enjoyment/
variety/lots of water for hydration of body and
easier 'elimination'.

The obvious suspects to avoid are:

wheat	rye	barley	dairy	coffee
MSG	fatty foods	red meat	fizzy drinks	tobacco
sugar	onions	chemicals	strong spices	alcohol

Some general steps you can take to help minimise symptoms and get your gut back to a state of well being:

HABITS	LIQUIDS
Eat at regular times or graze.	Drink 8 cups of water daily. In addition to hydrating and keeping healthy every single organ in your body, it also helps to keep faeces soft and easy to eliminate.
Don't leave long gaps between meals.	
Take your time, chew your food.	
Avoid chewing gum [Sorbitol an artificial sweetener]. Suck on a peppermint [sugar free] instead.	Cut back or eliminate coffee/tea or any caffeinated or carbonated drinks and alcohol.
FOOD	
Lightly cooked veggies can be easier on the gut than raw.	Be sensible about high fibre foods and fresh fruit – not too much, nor too little.
Lactose [sugar found in milk products] intolerance can be a problem. Experiment with eliminating milk.	Oats and Linseed can be excellent to decrease wind and bloating.
Go easy on fatty/fried foods.	Eat fish 3–4 times a week. Containing omega 3 fatty acids that can improve the digestive tract by stabilising the cell walls and reducing inflammation.
Some yogurts have probiotics that can help overall digestive health. Be careful if you are intolerant to dairy.	

LIFESTYLE	
Give up smoking – *I did it and can send you a free little advice sheet on what I did that may help you.* Posture – sit/stand up straight so that the organs have a little more space.	Exercise regularly – a good brisk daily 20 minute walk. Get enough sleep. Try and lose your excess weight.

☐ Drink a glass of warm water with a squeeze of lemon and a dash of salt before meals. This mixture naturally acts like the hydrochloric acid found in your stomach, it will help to remove excess bile from your liver and aid in the breakdown of food, improving digestion.

☐ Eat fresh papaya for dessert, a healthy and delicious fruit that is known for its powerful digestive enzymes. Eating a small portion of papaya after a meal will add to your body's natural and healthy enzymes and help it break down food

☐ Chew your food well, as saliva is the number one agent in food breakdown and digestion. For the next few days try slowing down, put your knife and fork down between mouthfuls, double the amount of times you normally chew. Your entire digestive system will benefit.

☐ Never eat more food than you can hold in both hands and try to leave at least 4 hours between meals. Eating excessively means partially undigested food reaches your colon, blocking the intestinal tract and disrupting the natural process of digestion.

☐ When you have time, begin the day with a warm oil massage, during which you apply gentle pressure over your abdomen in a clockwise motion.

☐ Don't consume too many cold drinks and food. Warmth stimulates digestion, while cold stifles digestion. In fact, drink a warm glass of water every morning. Put some lemon and honey in the water.

☐ Try peppermint oil for painful gas and bloating, and eat ginger for occasional nausea. I have a little bottle of organic peppermint oil in my bag and a dab on my tongue not only freshens the breath it also helps settle the digestion.

☐ Eat regular meals, planning your largest meal for the middle of the day between 12 p.m. and 2 p.m. Your last meal should be light and should be at least 2 hours before bedtime.

☐ Enjoy your meals while sitting. Mealtime should not be rushed or done on the go. Rest for a few minutes after finishing your meal.

☐ At night, drink a warm glass of milk [soya, if you are intolerant to lactose], spice with cinnamon and nutmeg.

☐ In addition to processed, avoid excessively hot and spicy foods and explore foods that are naturally cooling, that can help reduce any inflammation that may be present in the body and can be the cause of myriad problems. Such a diet may feel a little bland at first, but you will get used to it and your digestive tract will thank you for avoiding those extra hot vindaloos!

But how do you *really* fine tune your diet so that you are eating only the foods that really support your digestion rather than sabotage it?

1.   Energy test food[9] to determine what suits your body chemistry

2.   Elimination/observation to determine the same

Learning to Energy Test is fun and you will find over the years it can be an invaluable 'digestive aid'.

WHAT IS ENERGY TESTING?

This fascinating natural healthcare tool was originally developed, in the early 60s, in the field of Applied Kinesiology[10] by Dr George Goodheart a chiropractic physician from Detroit, and later expanded by various teachers, including: Touch for Health [John F. Thie D.C.] and Donna Eden [Eden Energy Medicine]. It was, and still is, a technique employed, by some dentists, chiropractors,

---

[9] I have a DVD available or go on YOU TUBE and tap in Madison King food testing and a couple of clips come up that you   may find useful; they are also on my site: www.midlifegoddess.ning.com

[10] The actual word Kinesiology comes from the Greek word KINESIS, which means motion. Applied Kinesiology was the name given by its inventor, Dr George Goodheart, to the system of applying muscle testing diagnostically and therapeutically to different aspects of healthcare.

physiotherapists, osteopaths, naturopaths, homeopaths and certain doctors.

Energy testing measures the integrity, efficiency and quality of the flow of energy through a particular muscle. It is not about how strong you or your friend are, it is about how well the energy is flowing through the muscle, its neurological response and ability to 'lock.

In kinesiology, there are over forty muscles one can test. For pure ease and simplicity, I have selected just two tests for use with friends and family, along with some self-testing techniques.

Energy testing enables us to access the body in a language that is easy to understand. The body can reveal to us, via the test of applying and resisting pressure on the muscle, if something strengthens or weakens it. It is truly that simple. Of course, nuances have been developed and it has become and 'art and science'. However, for our purposes, we are simply testing the body's reaction to a particular food or drink. This reaction will obviously impact on the entire digestive system.

The basic principle is that when a food is introduced into the body's energy field it will affect that field and therefore the body. If it is a food that the body cannot easily metabolise; it will result in a temporary weakness in the energy running through the body and the muscle being tested.

Conversely, food that suits the body's chemical makeup and that the body finds easier to metabolise, will strengthen it.

So, if a muscle can easily resist the pressure, if it remains unmoveable and strong, that is a positive result. If it either goes 'spongy' or totally weak that constitutes a negative result. We are assessing the quality of the muscle response in relation to a 'challenge' such as a food substance.

Please believe me when I say, that with a little practise, anyone and everyone can do these tests. I am not special; it is neither magic nor trickery. It is a practical bio-feedback tool to help you tune in to your body's needs. Use it with confidence on your children, spouse and friends.

Before we start, let's go through a few preliminaries…

- People don't like the unknown. Explain to your friend what you will be doing, stressing that it is a simple, quick, natural and organic technique, there is no pain involved.

- Reassure them that if a muscle is 'weak' it only means that the food being tested stresses their body, nothing more sinister.

- Make sure they have no injuries or problems that might get in the way of the test. Obviously avoid testing a muscle that is injured or weak for any reason. An accurate result will not be achieved from a shoulder that was dislocated last month!

- Neither of you should view this as a competition of strength.

- Check their posture is relaxed yet standing straight and nothing is crossed.

- Remind them that BREATHING normally is essential throughout – do not hold your breath.

- Don't try and second guess the test. Be objective and ready to embrace the truth!

- Common sense dictates that the tests will not be accurate if you have taken recreational drugs or alcohol!

- Dehydration can affect the test so both of you drink a glass of water beforehand.

- Remove any jewellery that may get in the way, watch, bangles etc.

Foods can be tested in their natural state, which for fruit etc., is very easy; there is no problem holding a banana or apple against your body. However, if the sample is messy, e.g. butter, put it [about a teaspoonful] in a clean glass jar or paper napkin. Normally neither of these materials weakens the body whereas using plastic packaging can deliver a weak test in itself. If you are in any doubt at all, just hold the substance in your hand and if you get mucky, wash the hand afterwards.

- Hold the food against the Solar Plexus, cheek or navel.

- Allow a couple of seconds for the body to register and absorb the sample's energy.

Testing is very much of the moment, a present tense. It is not a response of yesterday or tomorrow but very much on now, today. Reflect that in your thinking. Bring all your attention to what you are doing. So, put all expectations aside, remember one man's meat is another man's poison – take a deep breath and get started.

> *Whether testing for yourself or another person, always set as an objective that you SEEK THE TRUTH. What you do subsequently with that truth is entirely your choice.*

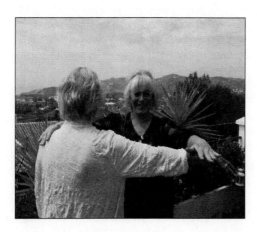

TECHNIQUE I

GENERAL INDICATOR MUSCLE

[Pectoralis major clavicular]

- Your friend stands up straight, unclenched and relaxed, with feet apart. [If necessary, the test can be done sitting]. Ask her to hold the food sample against her solar plexus, take a deep breath and be centred.

- Left arm [or right] is held out at a right angle to the body and parallel to the floor – this isolates the muscle, see position in photo.

- Check hand is *not* clenched into a fist – fingers should be straight.

- Stand in front of your friend, not too close, with your right hand, palm flat and facing downwards and fingers extended – resting on your friend's raised arm, on the forearm near the wrist joint. [shoulder side of the wrist].

- The left hand can rest gently on her shoulder.

- Demonstrate the range of movement – so that she is confident in what is about to happen. *You are interested in the first couple of inches* of that range, not everyone's arm drops all the way down to their hip. It might be that a 'spongy' response is all that is felt, but that is enough to indicate a weak result.

- Tell her to 'HOLD' – wait half a second, while her brain registers the command and then apply pressure for 2 seconds – gently, no jerking movements.

- What happened? If it locks and stays in position easily it means that it is testing STRONG.

- However, if it is spongy, or falls all the way down then that is a WEAK test.

If it is the first time testing, it is a good idea to check that the person is testing correctly. You do this by the following procedure:

> *Weaken them by running the palm of your hand backwards along the Central meridian[11] [down the centre of their torso].*
>
> *TEST – it should be weak i.e. the arm will go down or be spongy. Now run your palm up along the flow of Central [up the centre of the torso].*
> *TEST - it should be strong.*
> *This gives you a feel of their individual range and confirms they are testing correctly.*

NB – by bringing the outstretched arm towards the centre a little, it is possible to do this test on yourself – try it and see. If it doesn't feel right, there are some other self testing options below.

"Kinesiology is based on the fact that the body language never lies. Sometimes we do not understand what the body is trying to tell us, but that does not change the fact that the body is constantly expressing externally what is going on internally."

Sheldon Deal, DC, ND

---

[11] Tracing backwards on any channel of energy will weaken the body. Central runs up the body, so tracing down the body is against the flow and will weaken the person. At the end of the test, always ensure you trace upwards to leave the person strong.

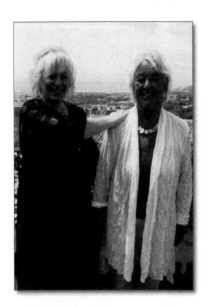

TECHNIQUE II

THE LATISSIMUS DORSI

[Spleen test]

This is an excellent alternative to the general indicator muscle [technique I], when testing foods, as it is directly associated with the Spleen and therefore involved in the metabolism of food.

Try them both [testing techniques I and II] and see which one you prefer.

The muscle used in this particular test sits under the shoulder on the side of the back and holds the shoulder down and helps keep the back straight.

Test with the arm straight down at the side, wrist turned back with thumb alongside the thigh and palm facing backwards. Some therapists use the back of the hand against the thigh, slightly more rotation. See which you prefer. Place the food sample against the person's solar plexus.

It is absolutely essential that the elbow of the arm being tested is straight. You can even pull down a little on the wrist to make sure the arm does not bend] and the torso does not move.

Put your open hand along the thumb side of her arm, just above the wrist. It is a matter of personal style and preference as to whether you come from back to front [as shown in this picture] or from front to back.

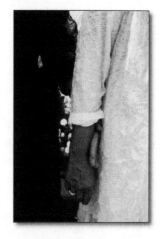

Now, say 'hold', wait a second for the brain to register the command before attempting to pull the arm straight outward away from her body. Your friend will resist the pull when you say 'hold'.

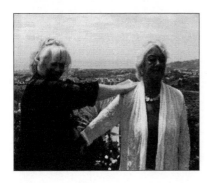

The same theory applies; if the arm pulls away easily it is a WEAK result. If it stays put firmly it is a STRONG result.

MY TOP TEN TIPS FOR
A SUCCESSFUL TEST

I have been energy testing for over twenty years now and the one thing I have learnt over those years is that everyone is different; we all develop our own unique style of testing – *it is intention and focus that is critical to accuracy*. Most of all, relax and have fun if you are learning to test – the more stressed you are, the more you think you 'can't do it', the more you doubt yourself and the test – the less accurate you will be. I personally was the world's worst tester when I was learning with Donna Eden until one day she told me to lighten up, enjoy it and have fun – I did and now I am pretty good at it! I reiterate: that does not make me special – anyone: male, female or child can test and test well.

This are some basic tips that may help you:

1. It is a good safeguard against dehydration to drink a glass of water five minutes before the test. Dehydration can adversely affect testing

2. Do not stand too close; keep a comfortable distance when testing.

3. Remove any jewellery or watch that may get in the way. Don't get too near to electrical equipment e.g. television or computer. Try and use samples free from plastic packaging

4. Gently tap on the bone between the breasts [over the Thymus gland] to put your friend into

a temporary state of balance. Do at the start of each test.

5. Both of you 'set the intention' that this will be an open and honest dialogue with the body. Sometimes food testing can be highly emotional – a chocoholic will find it impossible not to try and influence the chocolate test. Get round this by saying that you seek the truth in the test. What you do with that truth once you have it is entirely your choice.

6. Take a deep breath, relax and enjoy it BUT don't look into each other's eyes and don't smile [a smile literally has the power to strengthen your energy and interfere with the test].

7. Ensure neither of you hold your breath during the test.

8. Don't encircle her wrist and make sure she does not clench hers.

9. Leave egos outside the room [this is not a competition of strength] and avoid any jerky movements when testing. By exerting pressure gradually, you can be more sensitive to the response. This is particularly important if you have a person who does not show a greatly marked difference. i.e. her arm does not lower a lot.

10. Don't push down too hard for too long – anybody's arm will get spongy if you hang of it for 30 seconds! A second or two is sufficient to assess the reaction.

HOW TO TEST YOURSELF

There is not always someone available to test you when you have to make a decision on whether to buy/eat a specific food. No problem, here are some self testing techniques that offer a perfect solution. I suggest you try each of them and see which one you find the most effective, comfortable and the easiest, then stick with that one and practise, practise, practise.

It has to be said you can influence these tests if you choose to. Be sure that you are feeling as objective and neutral as possible. Tell yourself you are seeking the truth, any interference would only be self sabotage.

THE PENDULUM TEST

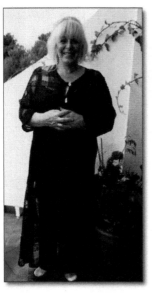

You will be using your body as a pendulum: stand, barefoot if possible, feet solidly on the floor, not too far apart, knees unlocked, take a deep breath, set the intention that you want an honest dialogue with yourself [easy to cheat].

Place one hand over your solar plexus and the other hand over the first. Doesn't matter which hand goes on top of the other.

Tuck your elbows into your sides.

Close your eyes and say *"my name is Minnie Mouse"*. Now, does your body sway forward or backward?

Repeat the test but this time saying *"my name is [your name]"* – what happens?

Normally the body will sway forward toward the truth or a substance that is strong/positive and easily metabolised and backward .i.e. away from one that is weak/negative, does not suit the body chemistry, or an untruth.

It will either be attracted or repelled. You will sway forward or backward.

However, rules are always made to be broken and some people buck this trend. You may even vary occasionally. By using the Minnie Mouse test you can establish your personal weak and strong sway for that day.

WITH FOODS

Simply hold the sample against the solar plexus or navel and see in which direction you sway.
Normally a forward sway indicates your body will tolerate that food and a backward sway that it is better to eliminate the food from your diet, at least for ten days and observe how you feel.

THE STICK TEST

The stick test was shown to me by Dr Michael Burt ND.[12] It is so discreet it can be used anywhere, anytime. In fact, a friend of mine who has been using it for years, can test the menu at any restaurant she visits, using this technique.

Nobody realises she is selecting the healthy choice for her body, in fact nobody knows she is doing it as she does it under the table, out of sight.

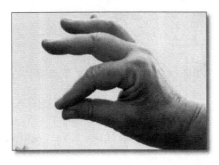

Centre yourself and take a deep breath, relax and rub the pads your index finger and thumb together, naturally, no real pressure. Now, as before, say "my name is Minnie Mouse" and observe what happens, do the fingers slide together more easily, or do they feel a little more 'sticky'? Repeat using your own name and observe what happens.

If you feel a marked difference, then this is a great test for you to practise as it is so easy and unobtrusive. Normally sliding more easily indicates a positive and feeling more friction, a certain 'stickiness' indicates a negative.

With food just hold the sample against your body and test.

---

[12] A truly remarkable naturopath in London – www.brabandhouseclinic.co.uk

THE QUAD TEST

Testing the quadriceps muscle is not quite as convenient, but it is easy and reliable: sit straight on a chair, with feet firmly planted on the ground in front, the chair should neither be too high nor too low.

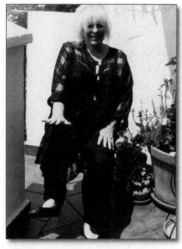

Place the food sample against your solar plexus or navel.

Lift one leg slightly off the chair. Now, with the heel of your hand, press down on that knee, while the knee resists.

If the leg stays locked take it as a strong result, your body can easily metabolise that food, it is not weakening it.

However, if the leg goes down easily then it is a weak result and it would be best to reduce or eliminate that particular food.

THE DUMBBELL TEST

Go to a sports store and head for the weightlifting section. Find a dumbbell that you can hold out in front of you with effort.

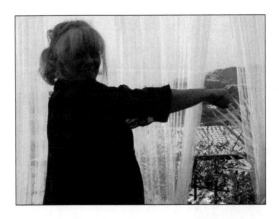

Hold it out and think a happy, vibrant thought[13] – does it feel easier to hold? Now think of something negative or depressing – is it now hard to hold? You need to select the weight that gives you this result.

A client of mine had a great idea: she had a pretty little wicker basket [with handle] into which she would put pebbles from the beach until she got exactly the right weight. If you didn't have a beach nearby you could use small bottles of water.

Place the 'weight' on a shelf at shoulder height. Hold a sugar cube in one hand. Stand in front of it and with other hand try to lift it. The energy of the sugar cube will affect the energy running through the muscle and it should be difficult to lift. Repeat with something you know your body likes, or say

---

[13] Thoughts generate subtle energies that affect our bodies. We can use this to our advantage in gauging the weight of the dumbbell but of course it has far reaching implications – don't harbour toxic thoughts or you will be weakening your body.

your name [my name is ....] and it should be easy to lift, thus indicating a strong test.

You then repeat the test using your food sample/s.

Because dumbbells exert a steady pressure downward [gravity], they provide a reasonably objective testing technique. It is important that you find the correct weight. Too light, or too heavy will reduce accuracy.

If you do not have a suitable shelf available, simply hold the weight by your side and see if you can pull the arm away from the body [this is the same principle as Technique II].

So all you have to do is to decide your test of choice and then test all your foods, go through your kitchen testing everything, go round supermarkets testing things. [I use the pendulum test a lot and I am sure the security guards are bewildered by what I am doing!]

You will then compile your personalised lists of foods you can eat and foods you cannot. Obviously professional food testing is a little more probing but this basic yes/no method is still effective. It is probably only confirming what you already know, or suspected.

I suggest you aim to eliminate foods that weaken you during the next 6 weeks. Even after just ten days you will begin to feel the benefit as your system begins to detox. At the end of 6 weeks take a step back and objectively measure what improvements you may experience: weight loss? Less stiffness? Reduced bloating? Healthier skin? Less moodiness?

You then retest to see if you can now slowly reintroduce some of the 'forbidden' foods back into your diet – see below.

The Observation Way

I am a devotee of energy testing foods but I am also realistic and aware that no one technique is suitable for everyone. If you do not feel comfortable testing yourself or being tested, there is another option. It takes a little longer but is effective. I call it the OBSERVATION method and there are two ways of doing it:

- **ALL OR NOTHING** – If you are feeling motivated the first version of this method is to eliminate: wheat, dairy, sugar and junk food [especially foods you crave], for **ten days** and then slowly reintroduce each one, observing how your body reacts. It is vital that you are honest and discerning in your observation and evaluation. In this way, you will recognise the foods that nurture you and the foods that stress you.

- **SLOW AND GENTLE** – if it seems too hard to eliminate all the above, honour your mindset, there is no right or wrong way, just the way that suits you. Try a slower approach

Days 1–10	Eliminate all wheat from your diet – scan labels.
Days 11–21	Eliminate all dairy.
Days 22–32	Eliminate all sugar – scan labels.
Days 33–43	Eliminate those foods that you crave, that you eat every day, or in excess, e.g. diet sodas, chemical rich foods.

At the end of each ten day period, observe how you look and feel, it will give you an indication of that food's effect on your body. If, at the end of the 43 days, you decide to eat the food again, carefully observe how your body reacts. It will give you the vital clues as to what foods you should be eliminating on a longer term basis. So the messages are clear, make sure you only reintroduce things one at a time; otherwise you will not know what is, or is not, causing a reaction.

A DIGESTIVE DIET

The human body is a complex biochemical miracle. By identifying foods with a chemical makeup that resonates well with your own personal body chemistry, you will be able to formulate a way of eating that matches your body to perfection, one that will strengthen and support it rather than weaken and sabotage it, ultimately leading to disease. You can eat a diet that is kind to your digestion, reducing the stress and damage that can be caused by a chemically rich and nutritionally bankrupt diet that is so favoured by the West.

'The proof of the pudding is in the eating', as my mother often reminds me. So eat this way for 6 weeks. That is to say, only eat those foods and drinks that test strong for you and eliminating totally those that test weak. It is as simple as that, eating only those foods that energise and support your body systems.

If you find you have to eliminate 3 or 4 of your favourite foods, honour your personality: are you an all or nothing person? Then eliminate them all at the same time. If however, you are more of a slow and steady person, eliminate them one at a time. Neither way is right nor wrong, it is a matter of what fits your personality type.

IT'S ONLY FOR 6 WEEKS!

a) Okay, so let's get real, it may not be possible to be 100% perfect 100% of the time, but do the best you can, don't give up – as Bob Hoskins said in Maid in Manhattan: *"What defines you is not that you fall, but how quickly you get up"* So, if you have a little binge-out. Get up, brush yourself down and start again straight away, don't beat yourself up, it's done, over – look forward positively.

b) If you do binge-out – do it in style and above all, enjoy it! Eat with joy, not with guilt. [Joy enhances the body's ability to metabolise the food, whereas guilt decreases that ability].

c) At the same time, introduce some of the other ideas in this little book; such as drinking lots of water, walking, getting more sleep.

d) After 6 weeks – retest, most foods will now test strong, but there may be a couple that still test weak – these are the ones you will have to be careful with in the future.

e) The foods that now test strong, you may reintroduce on a rotation basis, carefully observing the effect they have on your body.

LONG TERM STRATEGY

Take elements from the 6-week plan that you feel worked for you and integrate them into your daily life. Begin to create new healthier habits. Keep on with the food testing, test test test – after a while you will begin to develop a very clear intuition of what benefits your body and what does not. Your new found channel of communication with your body will flourish and you will be able to assess foods accurately at all times. You will be able to eat most foods, in moderation, probably on a rotational basis. Eating for energy will become second nature to you.

CREATING NEW HABITS

You have your list of foods, what are you going to do now?

- First of all, don't panic, don't sit there thinking, *"what on earth can I eat? oh woe is me!"* Rise to the challenge, swap old habits for new and feel the difference it makes.

- Get creative, buy a new healthy cookbook, there are many on the market. Use the internet, Google wheat free cooking, dairy free cooking etc., and see what inspiration comes up!

- Get organised, plan your menu, make a shopping list and ensure your kitchen is full of great foods that you can eat. You should never be hungry, there must always be something you can eat and enjoy, easy to hand.

- Clutter clear the kitchen of all foods that are prohibited for the next six weeks.

- Stock the fridge with great things, indulge in some expensive treats that suit your chemistry [mine are prawns, watermelon, melon, mango, raspberries and goats cheese].

- Buy quality, fresh or organic if possible.

- Become a label reader, we all fall foul of clever advertising and marketing, something that appears so healthy can have some sinister ingredients when you study the label.

- Chew chew chew your food – no 'mindless munching' – eating must be conscious and enjoyed with all the senses. Chewing is good for two reasons, firstly it initiates digestion and if the food in your mouth is well broken down before it is swallowed, it is processed more easily as it transits through the digestive tract. Secondly, you will eat less, as you will be eating more slowly and your satiety point will kick in before you overeat.

- Never eat in a stressful situation such as listening to the TV news or having an argument. Also I would suggest you don't chew gum, it makes the body think you are going to swallow food and it produces digestive juices in anticipation; when no food arrives, those juices can, over time, cause damage to the stomach's lining.

- Don't eat on the hoof. Eating should be a 'sacred ritual' or one at least that you are conscious of. Eat slowly, put your knife and fork down between mouthfuls, and don't let the savage pig run wild.

- Check portion sizes, a fist full of each food is a good benchmark. I am a girl with a healthy appetite, some might say a savage pig resides within me, so I try to discipline myself on portion size, if not, I end up eating healthy food, yes, but a portion size to suit an 18 year old 6'4" rugby player.

- Drink lots of water – backache/hunger is often a symptom of thirst.

- Consider setting yourself an eating curfew, so that you are not consuming large heavy meals late at night, just before you go to bed. Of course, it is not always possible to avoid this, but keep such meals to a minimum.

- Consider 'grazing' – i.e. small amounts of food, frequently eaten, as opposed to 3 square meals a day. There is an argument that this stimulates the metabolism. Does it fit into your lifestyle? Try it and see how you feel.

- At the risk of repeating myself, but it is an important point: Honour your personality – all or nothing [cut out everything all at once] or slow and gentle [one thing a week] – there is no wrong or right way, it has to be the way to suit you.

- Keep reminding yourself that it is not forever, only 6 weeks and there will be a huge feedback on your investment!

- Remember that there is a life beyond food, go out and live it.

- You are not denying your body anything you are GIVING it a gift.

- Cultivate a positive attitude – you are <u>not</u> going to be a victim anymore, you are taking control, you are reclaiming your life. Time and energy that can be spent on more enjoyable pursuits.

- You may have a few detox symptoms, such as bad breath, headache or even spots, as your body rids itself of numerous toxic gremlins, but they will quickly pass. Don't be discouraged. Drink lots of water to help flush the toxins out, along with a Milk Thistle supplement to support your Liver through this busy time. However, if they go on for more than a few days, consult your natural healthcare practitioner, you may have Candida, which when it is starved, can produce strong detox symptoms for some time.

- In addition to a happier digestive system, the benefits of energy foods that suit your own personal body chemistry include:
    - Health, vitality and stamina
    - Loss of excess weight
    - Less bloating
    - Reduction of fatigue
    - Less toxins to pollute the body
    - Less stress to overload the systems
    - Improved mood and more 'joy in life'
    - You glass seems to be half full not half empty
    - Improved sleep patterns
    - Improved body functions
    - Improved complexion

You will feel better on all levels that can be measured; as you are effectively giving your body a helping hand, giving it a chance to cope with the changing environment we find ourselves in, bringing it back from frontline confrontation with the contemporary predators of stress and pollution.

At this point, I want to share with you a little extra technique taught to me by John Thie [Touch for Health]. When I saw it, my eyes must have lit up as the little piggy inside me saw a way of indulging the savage pig, but JT stressed, looking me straight in the eye, that this was not to be abused but could be used occasionally to limit damage...

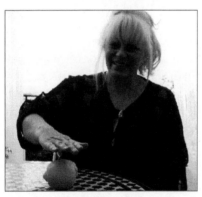

Bless Your Food

To neutralise toxic gremlins and make the food less harmful to your body. Sit in front of it quietly and place your left hand about a foot above the food, slowly circle in an anticlockwise direction, imagining all the toxic gremlins being drawn out of the food. Stop and shake off this hand to the floor. Now raise your right hand a few inches above the food and make two or three circles in a clockwise direction, imagining light and nutrition entering the food. Now, eat and enjoy!

SUPPLEMENTATION

The following supplements can be helpful in your quest for digestive nirvana. Do not take them all, be discerning and select just one or two to try. If you are confident, energy test [in the health shop] to determine which ones/brands test strong for you. If in any doubt ask advice from shop staff or a nutritionist.[14] Normally organic brands are more efficient.

B Complex is excellent for our nervous system and also for the integrity and efficiency of the intestinal muscles.

VITAMIN C and QUERCETIN can act as antihistamines and are useful in reducing inflammation in the digestive tract. I have found Quercetin and Bromalin a powerful synergistic mix to bring down inflammation anywhere in the body – joints and even a tooth abscess responded well to splitting the capsules, mixing with a little olive oil and applying topically. This has no solid research behind it but has worked for me on several occasions – it certainly can do you no harm to try it.

---

[14] There are so many good health stores nowadays but if you do not have one locally, visit or call NUTRICENTRE. Based near Regents Park in London, I have used them for years and find the products they stock and their level of knowledge and helpfulness to be excellent http://www.nutricentre.com/ they do international delivery too www.bodykind.com is another site I have found, although not yet used, that seems backed with good quality supplements.

DIGESTIVE ENZYMES are produced naturally by your body, taking them as a supplement can be helpful.

There are three types of digestive enzymes:

1. To digest protein – proteolytic
2. To digest fat – lipases
3. To digest carbohydrates – amylases

CoQ10 can work synergistically with the enzymes, improving their efficiency. There is a lot of research being undertaken on CoQ10 especially in relation to the heart.

PROBIOTICS – such as acidophilus, have become very popular and have had a lot of publicity over the last decade; especially in relation to Candida [see Coping with Candida in the Essential series]. Those little probiotic drinks and yoghurts are now consumed by over 2 million of us! With so much interest, research is rife and suggests that probiotics could help a wider range of problems than just the gut.

Briefly, they are good, friendly bacteria needed for a healthy, friendly flora balance in the gut. The balance can be disturbed by external influences such as stress, drugs, antibiotics etc. They are normally 'live' and should be kept in a fridge once opened. You may need a bit more than a yoghurt 'shot', go for a product that contains at least Lactobacillus acidophilus and Bifidobacterium. If you are prescribed antibiotics take a probiotic product at the same time.

I took them when I travelled in North Africa, along with colloidal silver, they really helped me resist all those little bugs and germs that were just dying to attack my body. They definitely helped protect my gut.

So, what else do they do? They: aid digestion; maximise the absorption of nutrients through the intestinal wall and can aid efficient peristalsis and therefore elimination. They even have the potential to boost your immune system.

SLIPPERY ELM – is a North American herb and comes from the inner bark of the elm tree. It has been used for many years, by the Native American Indians for digestive healing. Its prime benefit is its ability to sooth an irritated gut and relieve minor pain and inflammation, so particularly useful when dealing with IBS.

Don't take this herb if you are pregnant

ACID ALKALINE BALANCE – is important for digestive health, as it is for all systems in the body. There are many products on the market that help maintain a healthy pH balance which can be upset by stress and diet. If you suspect you are too acidic, revise your diet to eliminate some of the obviously acid forming foods: coffee, processed or chemically rich foods, meat, alcohol, sugar, salt and more.

I have found a useful way of regaining a healthy pH balance is to use alkalising drops: simply add a few drops to your water.

BARLEY GRASS is a good alkalising supplement too.

CHLORELLA is one of today's 'super foods' – a green algae that grows in freshwater ponds in the Far East, Australia and North America. New Japanese research suggests it aids digestion and relieves IBS. It is also protein packed – containing twice as much as spinach and is power packed with nine essential amino acids, vitamins and minerals.

ALOE VERA – renowned for calming an irritated digestive tract. It can be taken as a juice or tablet and can even be applied topically for burns and skin problems. It is anti-inflammatory and has the ability to rebuild balance in the digestive tract by soothing inflammation, removing harmful bacteria and toxic waste

APPLE CIDER VINEGAR 3 or 4 teaspoons of a good quality organic apple cider vinegar in a medium sized glass of warm water with a touch of honey and slice of lemon every morning, can help digestion, bowel regularity, removal of toxins and maintain pH levels in the body. The brand Braggs is a good one. [15]

CAPRILYIC ACID helps maintain a healthy balance of intestinal flora. It comes from the natural oils of the palm and coconut. It is said to be antibacterial, viral and fungal. A powerful tool in the fight against Candida;[16] it is also excellent in reducing intestinal inflammation, it is being researched in the treatment of Crohn's Disease. Solgar Caprilyic Acid is available online from the Nutricentre in London. www.nutricentre.com

---

[15] www.bragg.com
[16] See Coping with Candida, part of the Essential Series

GINGER – Cultures throughout the planet and the centuries have realised the health helper that ginger can be. Another good anti inflammatory agent, ginger can help relieve tummy ache, nausea, sickness and diarrhoea. If you don't like the taste, use a supplement. I personally love it and will add it to many of my stews, stir fries, soups etc.

Try this herbal mix I use a lot, just for the pleasure of the taste, let alone the benefits to my digestion.

- Sliced ginger
- Melissa leaves
- Crushed cardamon seeds
- Mint leaves
- Honey

Mix all the ingredients above in hot water in a saucepan and heat, just off the boil, simmering for a few minutes. Quantities, experiment to find your taste. Let it steep and then drink hot or cold. I tend to make a litre or two at a time; it will keep in the fridge for a few days.

Add anise or fennel to minimise bloating and gas.

Add dill to lessen indigestion and heartburn.

PEPPERMINT is another one from our grannies' medicine chest. The Harvard Medical School report that 75% of patients in an Italian study, who took peppermint oil capsules for 4 weeks had a major reduction in their IBS symptoms [compared to 38% of those who took a placebo]. One explanation is that the oil can relax the intestinal walls.

CAMOMILE – I spend a lot of time in Southern Spain where the locals drink Camomile [manzanilla] tea to aid digestion. Science is also showing an interest in the benefits of this plant. London Imperial College conducted research into its ability to ease muscle spasm and fight inflammation especially in the intestinal tract. Don't overdo Camomile if you are pregnant, it could ease your muscles a little too much.

ORAGANO. An effective anti-bacterial and anti-viral herb that also has antioxidant properties [preventing oxygen based damage to cell structures throughout the body]. Specific to the digestion is its anti-parasitic properties and others that ease indigestion.

Make an infusion to help abdominal muscle spasm.

PSYLLUM AND BENTONITE CLAY CLEANSE. This is a popular intestinal cleanse, that has been used for centuries in Europe, the cleanse helps remove excessive toxic waste and build up on the intestinal wall. It is obviously going to be better for our overall health if the intestines are clean from putrefied matter, bacteria, toxins and parasites. None of these therefore aren't going to be leaking back into the body and causing mischief and bowel movements become easier, regular and more efficient. Rehydration and efficient removal of waste is crucial for a healthy colon and therefore overall health.

Psyllium husks [the outer hull of the seeds of the Plantago plant] are mixed with water to create a 'gelatine-like' substance. It helps hydrate and soften the faeces and lubricates evacuation. It is bulky and helps 'push' the faeces along the colon.

Bentonite Clay is a highly absorbent natural clay that can absorb and bind toxins in the intestinal tract and then eliminate with the faeces.

The general recipe is:

- 1 heaped teaspoon of Psyllium husks
- 1 teaspoon of Bentonite clay power
- 8 oz plain water

Mix together briskly and drink immediately, before it thickens

Follow with a glass of plain water [8oz min]

Do twice daily; taken between meals and at least 2 hours before or after taking supplements or medications. Drink extra warm water, with or without lemon juice.

Do whenever you feel sluggish, heavy, bloated or constipated.

The cleanse can be for however long you feel it appropriate: a couple of days or an entire week.

There are some interesting products such as Lepicol on the market today, that combines fibre and probiotics and can be useful in cleansing the gut.

COLLOIDAL SILVER – I travelled extensively in Egypt and Morocco. I always took my little bottle of colloidal silver and even though I ate from street vendors and with tribes in the desert – I never got sick. I am not suggesting you throw commonsense to the winds but I am suggesting that colloidal silver kept me safe during my travels. Sadly it is now illegal in Europe [as from January 2010] but is freely available in the USA.

FLOWER ESSENCES

There are so many flower essences available now. Because of space, I am going to focus on two of my favourite brands: Australian Bush Flower Essences[17] and Healing Herbs.[18]

Here are a few for you to consider. First the Australian Bush Flower Essences:

BLACK EYED SUSAN – a suitable antidote for the stresses of contemporary life: always on the go, rushing, multi tasking, taking on all the responsibility, not delegating, not being able to wind down. Not allowing time for their digestive juices to do their job – often eating on the hoof, grabbing and gulping their food. Because of being in a rush their food choices will be poor.

If your nervous system is busy dealing with stress it will be sending the blood away from the stomach, thus diminishing its digestive ability. Black eyed Susan will help you get a better balance and perceptive and reduce your stress response, thus aiding stress-related digestive problems.

PAW PAW when you feel in overwhelm, drowning under the load and not able to cope with it all. The fruit itself contains Papain and helps most types of digestive problems: the essence, combined with CROWEA, which is wonderful for worry, really helps disperse the anxiety that can weaken the stomach when financial problems hit us, perhaps

---

[17] www.ausflowers.com.au
[18] www.healingherbs.co.uk

unemployment, having to face the unknown. Take this combination to lighten the anxiety and therefore to begin to see a way forward. **Crowea** is also helpful in regulating the acid: alkaline balance in the stomach.

PEACH FLOWERED TEA TREE is effective for treating Candida. [see my book Coping with Candida].

From Healing Herbs, try **Beech** if you feel you have difficulty focusing inward and digesting what is going on in your life.

ESSENTIAL OILS

These can be used in a good quality carrier oil [such as sweet almond or an organic olive oil] and massaged over the entire abdominal area. Always move in a clockwise direction, from the left hip, over to the right hip, then up under the right breast over to the left and down to the left hip again, this circle direction follows the natural transit of the intestines.

Choose from ones I have already discussed:

- Cardamon essential oil
- Roman Chamomile
- Lavender
- Ginger
- Peppermint

And also...

Black Pepper stimulates circulation [my personal favourite is to mix it with Sweet Marjoram] it is excellent for sluggish bowels. The herb itself can irritate the bowel, but the essential oil does not.

Sweet Fennel works well on constipation and stomach spasm. Avoid if you are pregnant.

Grapefruit – stimulates digestion and rounds out a blend with an uplifting note.

Hyssop – for indigestion and should be avoided during pregnancy.

Sweet Marjoram – for constipation, colic and flatulence.

Rosemary – a tonic for digestion.

CHAKRA BALANCE

The entire chakra system can be involved in digestive problems but the obvious two chakras to work on would be the 2nd chakra, right over the lower abdominal area and the 3rd one over the solar plexus area.

Let me share a few basic concepts about both with you. There will be an entire book on chakras but this will give you a flavour, a feel of these two and a simple way to bring calm and balance to them.

2ND **CHAKRA** — *is sometimes called the Womb or Sacral Chakra*

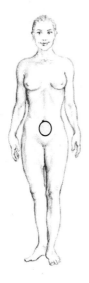

Located in the area between your navel and pubic bone, it is home to your GUT FEELING. Also to the 'butterflies' and any anxious 'churning' that can so often accompany stress and worry.

Take time to think about <u>*why*</u> your digestion may be less than perfect. Seldom is anything 'just' 100% physical, often there is an emotional connection underpinning the physical symptom.

- ☐ This chakra is the home of your natural child, your basic, innocent 'me/soul/self' before it becomes wounded by life

- ☐ It is the protected home of imagination and creativity. That actual womb carries the highest of all creation — a baby! If blocked — is your creativity blocked too, are you frustrated? Could this reflect in constipation?

- ☐ Be still and make contact with the pure innocent self contained in this Chakra. Get to know this 'self'. If you want to know why you came here to this planet at this time and what your purpose is: meditate on this chakra

- Don't try making any sense of things using this chakra. It does not house logical, linear thought – it is about surrendering to faith and trust

- This is the home of your natural healing abilities – your umbilical cord to the universal 'knowing'

- The 'hara' is located in the auric field between the 2nd and 3rd chakras. Many 'healers' will breathe and work from this energy centre.

- Associated with water, if this chakra shows weak for you, ask yourself a question: are you *'going with the flow'*? Am I letting go of things, people and situations to enable myself to move on?

3rd CHAKRA

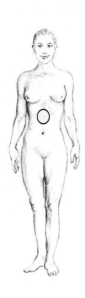

This is energetically where you grow up! Located in the solar plexus area, this is the home of self worth, identity, ego and fear. It is the *'power'* chakra and is where many of the negative emotions associated with the stress of everyday life are generated: discrimination, assertion, fear, anxiety, stress, grief, anger, resentment, guilt, calculation, and thinking, logic, related to needs of the ego, willpower, self determination, autonomy, cunningness and suspicion.

It can also affect our ability to take decisions; we all know that churning feeling when we have to make a decision that may affect the rest of our lives – pure stress.

- ☐ We can easily be ruled by this chakra in today's society
- ☐ The Solar Plexus is where identity and ego are built
- ☐ It also houses the feeling of '*this is who I am, this is who I want to be, this is how I want to be seen*'
- ☐ Find your mission/direction in life. Sometimes conflict with what we want to do and what we think we ought to do
- ☐ Parental influences and control issues are imprinted here
- ☐ The innocent self of the 2nd chakra moves into this chakra and is blown apart by the activity it finds here. Innocence is lost. It then begins to adapt to the pressures it encounters
- ☐ Affected by the Triple Warmer meridian which is in itself affected directly by stress and what it perceives to be 'survival' issues

As you can probably feel, just by reading that list, this is the chakra that can generate stress and in turn be hit by everyday stress, in a big way. Any digestive problems will benefit from a simple balancing technique. If you are not familiar with chakra balancing, I would ask you to just keep an open mind and try it, or even better, get your partner or friend to balance your chakra – you may be surprised at how good it feels and how effective it is.

SOLAR PLEXUS CRADLING[19]

If you feel your digestion responding to stress, try this simple exercise.

- Sit quietly and take some deep breaths.
- Rub your hands together and shake off.
- Place your hands over the 3rd chakra and cradle it, hold it gently and thank it for working so hard. Feel gratitude.
- Cradle and calm it as you would a baby.
- You might like to hold your favourite crystal against it or use sound, an essence or oil [described above].
- Be calming and kind to it. Today's society and its demands and pressures are a great burden to it. You are trying to convince it to let go a bit and not get caught up in the fear of it all, entice it to step off the merry go round for a while.

BELT FLOW

There is a flow off energy around the waist, called the Belt Flow. It can become stagnant and sluggish and begin to affect the organs below. It pays huge dividends to spend a few seconds making sure it is moving and therefore supporting rather than stifling the digestive organs.

---

[19] *With thanks to Anna Maria for her lovely drawing.*

- With fingers spread, circle the hands around the side of the body at the waist. Pull from the back of the body to the front and all the way across the belly and to the other side. Pull not only at the waist, but above and below it as well.

- Do this several times with some pressure and a lifting movement, alternating hands. Then firmly slide both hands down the leg on the side you are pulling toward and off the foot. Repeat on the other side of the body.

Also, when you are in the shower, with soapy hands imagine a belt around your waist and pull it apart one hand pulling up towards your head and the other down towards your feet, all around the entire waist area, creating space for energy to flow around your waist. Push in and pull up/down with some pressure, that is why doing it in the shower with soapy hands, makes it more comfortable to go deeper.

HANDS 'STIRRING THE SOUP'

A BASIC CHAKRA BALANCE

This is best done with a friend, but can be done on yourself

With your hand just away from the body, so not actually touching it, take a moment to connect in with your friend. They will be on their back.

Slowly start circling your left hand [or both hands if you prefer] in an anti-clockwise circle above the chakra. This is where you can really connect in with the energy and feel it moving under your hands, maybe even pushing your hands out and up.

[These are just guidelines, if you prefer to use the right hand then please do].

Feel the energy, where is it? What is it doing? Your hand is acting like a magnet and drawing out toxic/stagnant energy from the chakra. Keep circling until you feel a change in the energy. Visualise the energy coming up and out of the chakra.

How do you feel, do you have any thoughts or pictures coming into your mind that might be relevant? Doesn't matter if you don't but if you do – just observe them, don't analyse or judge. They can be discussed later.

Shake off your hands onto the floor, so the earth can take up the energy and transmute it.

Now circle your other hand [right or both] in a clockwise direction above the same chakra. This will harmonise the energy. Keep circling until you feel the energy is strong. Take as long as you need. Concentrate and remember to breathe.

If the energy feels particularly heavy – rock your friend gently backwards and forwards to help release it. Then turn them over so they are face down and rock the sacral area.

Normally we only need to work the front of the chakras – but if you feel the pull to do so, work the back of them too. I heard a wonderful theory a couple of years ago: you ask the angels to take away the 'rubbish being pulled out' –

Ask them, you have nothing to lose.

Trace relevant energy pathways

One of the simplest ways to remove harmful congestion and get energy flowing to the organs is to trace the pathways [meridians]. If you go either on my Facebook page [Madison's Medicine] or on You Tube there is a great video clip of Donna Eden tracing meridians. [I shall be posting one myself in 2014 – so take a look]. Some people find it easy to learn by watching. Others by listening, so for those just record the instructions below and play them back to yourself every day – after four or five days you will know the pathways.

SMALL INTESTINE

Start on the little fingernail, trace straight up the outside of the arm to the shoulder, drop back down on the shoulder blade and then come up to your cheekbone and straight back to the opening of the ear. Both sides are done. [This is also a good meridian to work if you have any shoulder problem].

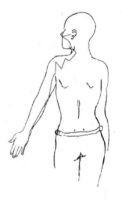

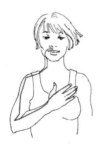

LARGE INTESTINE – start at the index fingernail and trace straight up the arm to the front of the shoulder. Continue up the neck to just beneath your nostril and go out to the flair of your nose – it always reminds me of Hercule Poirot's moustache. Do both sides.

GALLBLADDER – bring the fingertips of both hands to your temples. Drop back to the opening of your ears. Move fingers straight up about two inches then circle forward in a small loop and drop back behind the ears; go forward again over to your forehead, back over the crown of your head, and around your shoulders; leave your shoulders, take your hands to the sides of your rib cage, go forward on the rib cage, back on the waist, forward on the hips, straight down the sides of the legs and off the fourth toes

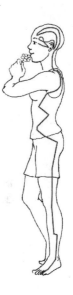

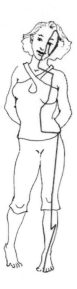

STOMACH – Place the fingertips of both hands beneath your eyes. Drop them down to your jawbone then circle up the outside of the face until you arrive on the forehead in line with your eyes. Move down through the eyes to the collarbone, move your hands outwards a little and down over each breast, keep going down, coming in at the waist a little, out at the hips, straight down each leg and off the toe next to the big toe.

[Did you know that if this toe is longer than your big toe, the Chinese believe you have a true 'appetite for life' – great leaders have this toe but so do 'holics' of any kind ... be warned you workaholics].

LIVER – I love tracing Liver as it is so easy and I can do both sides at the same time. Place fingers on the outside of each big toe nail [i.e. the side next to the second toe]. Now simply trace straight up the inside of the legs, coming out at the hips to go up the sides of the rib cage to about where your bra sits, then move into towards your centre line, ending in line with the nipples.

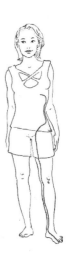

GETTING TO THE SOURCE

On each of the above pathways of energy there is one particular point that is like a mini reservoir of energy that constantly gets replenished. If you massage or work this point it will literally hyperlink energy direct to the organ in question.

The simplest way to work these points is to hold them and massage firmly, followed by tracing a tiny Figure 8 over them.

So where are these points: 2 are on the hands and 3 on the feet:-

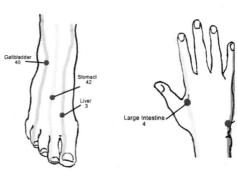

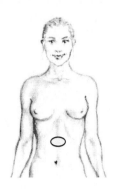

One other point you might find useful is located half way between the navel and the bottom of the breastbone. It is actually the point for the 'digestive 'system and is also what is called the Stomach Alarm Point. Work this point to stimulate the entire intestinal system.

Don't swallow your stress, anger or irritation

It is imperative that we don't continually internalise our stress, anger or irritation because eventually these emotions will cause problems such as gastric ulceration, literally *'eating itself with worry'.*

Equally it is important that we face, process and let go of anger, resentment or any hint of bitterness, be it outwardly or inwardly directed. If not, it can play havoc with our Liver and Gallbladder which can have a knock-on effect to almost every single system in our body. So important are these two organs that I am writing a whole book on the implications of having a grumpy gallbladder and livid liver – watch out for it in a few weeks.

So find a way of expelling your personal venom, perhaps blowing it away and out of your life – see the exercise earlier in the book. Maybe using an affirmation such as:

> **I now look at my anger,**
>
> **I love it,**
>
> **I learn from it**
>
> **And I let it go, easily and quickly.**
>
> **All is well.**

Special points to massage

There are key reflex points on the outside and inside of each thigh. When massaged firmly they stimulate the large and small intestines.

Easy to locate: imagine you are wearing a pair of trousers – where the inside and outside leg seams sit – there are the rows of points to work. Each point must be massaged firmly. They might be tender but persevere.

It doesn't matter what direction you massage in but if you are constipated, massaging from hip to knee will help loosen those bowels. If they are too loose already then work knee to hip.

A little tip: these will probably be a little painful [oh the British art of understatement] at first and your leg will automatically move away – to stop this, hold the other side of the leg and push in.

An added extra is to make an affirmation of your choice while massaging the points: for example...

> **I now release with ease all that needs to come out on both a physical and emotional level – all is well**

Houston and Illeocecal valves

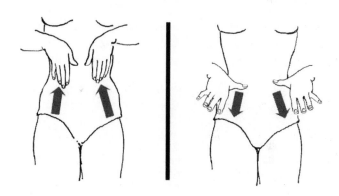

Do you feel tired, cranky, lethargic, hung-over? Are there dark circles under your eyes, is your skin telling a toxic tale? This is a simple technique to get you back on track. It can be used at any time, whenever you are feeling a wee bit toxic or your digestion is playing up.

It resets the Illeocecal Valve, which, located on the right hand side of the tum, is a one way valve that allows digested food to pass from the small to the large intestine for further processing. It stops waste materials from backing up into the small intestine [rather like a backed up sink drain] Simple, but when it goes wrong it can cause huge problems of toxicity in the body. What can cause it to go wrong? Dehydration, bad eating behaviours such as under chewing food, eating too quickly, eating the wrong foods: sodas, alcohol, caffeine, sugar etc., and of course, emotional stress of any kind.

Whether the valve is stuck open or closed you can use the same correction technique. Problems such as eczema, bronchitis, digestive disorders, lower backaches can all clear up after this valve's functioning is restored. Best done in the shower with soapy hands, resetting this valve can reap huge benefits and takes less than 30 seconds!

1. *Place the right hand on the right hip bone with the little finger at its inside edge. Your hand is now over the valve.*

2. *Place the left hand at the corresponding spot on the inside edge of the left hipbone. This is the houston valve, resetting both valves creates a symmetry between them.*

3. *Firmly massage in a circular motion and then slowly drag the fingers of each hand up six to seven inches with a deep inhalation. Keep the pressure of the drag as deep as you can.*

4. *Shake the energy off your fingers with the outbreath and return to the original position. Repeat about 4 times*

5. *End by dragging your fingers downward one time with pressure*

DRY SKIN BRUSHING

The Russians, Turks and Scandinavians have used this treatment for centuries.

Now you can benefit and brush your way to a beautiful body

Dry skin brushing could be your new best friend. It works on two levels: on the superficial, it will give you softer, smoother more velvety skin; on the 'inner', it will help detox and boost your immunity and is a quick and easy tool to stimulate your digestion and elimination.

Our bodies are living in a world they have not yet fully evolved into. Think of all the technological advances of the past eighty years that we live with in our daily life. Consider what is in the air that was not there 50 years ago: cell phone, radio, TV, Satellite a veritable host of EMFs [electromagnetic frequencies] polluting our lives and I won't even begin to go into how we self-pollute with sugar, alcohol, drugs, rubbish foods and chemicals... you get the general idea.

Normally the human body would have thousands of years to adapt to such changes but no, we have given ourselves less than a lifetime and our bodies, on the whole, are doing a miraculous job at coping BUT at a cost. Coping makes continual demands on our bodies – especially our digestion and after a while, albeit a few years, the digestive, immune and other systems begin to falter under such an unrelenting load, resulting in illness such as: arthritis, cancer, diabetes, skin problems, heart etc.

We cannot change the world we live in, but we can exert control over our own individual little universes... common sense changes such as: eating healthily, exercising more, drinking lots of water, positive attitude and also dry skin brushing all help support the body in its battle with the techno elements.

The lymphic system is like the body's housekeeper, some call it a garbage disposal. It comprises a vast, delicate network of vessels and nodes that filter, purify, cleanse and detox the entire body. Many of these vessels lie just under the skin and dry skin brushing will stimulate the entire system, purging toxins from the body. It also helps remove old dead skin cells, opening up the pores and increasing elimination. [The skin is the largest organ of the body and can eliminate up to 2lbs of waste daily.] Lung, Large Intestine and Kidney are the other primary detoxifiers and organs of elimination. A weakness in any one organ, forces the others to carry an increased workload which can in turn result in exhaustion and further inhibit the body's ability to get rid of harmful toxic waste. Daily dry skin brushing helps your skin remain vibrant and efficient so that organs are not stressed or overloaded.

It only takes a minute, do it a couple of times a day on dry skin *before* taking a shower, certainly before a workout as it opens pores and allows sweat to remove more waste.

For us 'ladies of a certain age', dry skin brushing is a godsend. Aging skin does not shed its outer layer of dead cells as efficiently as younger skin. The build-up of this outer skin layer accounts for the thick, dry, "leathery" look of older skin (along with too much sun exposure). Skin brushing exfoliates this layer. It also stimulates the oil glands, providing more moisture for older skin. Further good news is that it helps break down cellulite and tightens the skin and can improve muscle tone by stimulating the nerve endings which causes the individual muscle fibres to activate and move. It can help mobilise fat, stimulate hormone function, the nervous system and blood circulation in the underlying organs and connective tissue. Pretty good payback for a couple of minutes brushing a day.

Unlike blood, which has the heart to pump it around the body, the lymphatic system relies on movement, exercise and gravity for its circulation, so walk when you can, move the body, treat yourself to a massage to encourage the flow.

All you need for this technique is a **_soft_** bristle brush. They are normally set in wood, either circular to fit into the palm of your hand, or oval with a detachable handle. Do not get a hard one as that is more use for stimulating blood circulation, for lymph we need the softness of a baby!

A cunning trick is to use TWO BRUSHES, get a rhythm going and you will have done your entire body in no time at all.

Use a light pressure and brush, on dry skin, in long sweeping strokes.

The basic rule of direction is: imagine a belt around your waist, anything below that belt gets brushed into the groin and anything above the belt goes to the armpits.

On the legs, I suggest you start at the knee and brush up into the groin all around the thigh, then linger a little around the inside of the knee [lymph nodes are located here so the area can often feel tender].

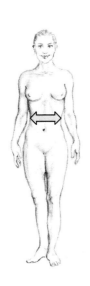

Now move down to the ankles and brush up to the knee all around the lower leg. Brush around the top of the foot, I studied the Vodder Lymphatic Drainage Technique [Austria] and they romantically call this area 'The Sea of Lymph'.

Proceed with long strokes from toe to groin. In this way, you are 'clearing' an area before brushing new lymph into it.

Move on to hands and arms, then back [this is where a brush with a detachable handle comes in useful], abdomen, shoulders and neck.

Now jump into the shower and get rid of all that dead skin: use an exfoliating sponge or cloth [Dermalogica do a great one] and if you can bear it, finish off with a cold blast of water. Dry with a rough towel, rub in some oil or cream and voila! ... you will feel invigorated and ready to start the day.

TIP 1 – to help prevent slack skin as you age or lose weight, massage and 'pinch' the skin. It will stimulate the circulation, feeding the tissue and encouraging elasticity in the skin.

Tip 2 – further stimulate lymphatic function by firmly massaging the neuro lymphatic reflex points located on the front of the shoulder, exactly where your arm would be 'sewn on' to the torso.

Tip 3 – stimulate the large and small lymphatic reflex points along the outside and inside of each thigh [described earlier in the book].

Clean your brush using soap and water once a week. After rinsing [maybe a drop of Tea Tree or Lavender essential oil in the rinse water], dry it in an open, sunny spot to prevent mildew.

Try it and see, after a couple of weeks you should begin to notice a difference, a lot less sluggish and your general immunity will improve. After three months you will definitely be an addict and begin to crave your daily 'brush off'.

A few words of caution... Even though you are working with soft bristles, your skin may feel a little tender or sensitive at first, be gentle and soon it will feel good. Obviously don't brush any broken or damaged skin. If the skin becomes red or irritated in any way, you are using too much pressure, ease off. Your skin will soon become used to the technique and will cease to be sensitive.

After several days of dry brushing, you may notice a gelatinous mucous material in your stools. Don't panic, this is a sign that the intestinal tract is renewing itself.

If you have cancer, serious skin problems or just feel a little uneasy about brushing, have a word with your doctor first.

Exercise and stretching

This is just common sense really – your digestion will improve greatly if you simply take a 20 minute brisk walk daily. Wear sensible shoes, don't carry a heavy handbag and walk on a flat and even surface. Walking gets everything moving.

Equally, if you are sitting at a desk all day your entire digestive system is constricted with a distinct lack of space for blood, liquids, waste, lymph and energy to move. Stand up, raise your hands above your head and arch your back a little, stretching out the entire front of your torso. Then stretch to the left and then to the right. Stretching doesn't have to be time consuming or complicated... 30 seconds every hour will work wonders. Put a post it note where you will see it and be reminded.

Be inventive or take a look at some of the myriad stretches available today in books and online.

Crystals

You can wear these as jewellery, carry in your pocket or bra [although make sure you don't lose them], tape it to your body; or simply lie still, breathing with the crystal on your abdomen.

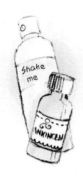

Crystals are powerful and if you are ever in doubt about wearing them on your body – here's a safe alternative. An extremely gentle way of using crystal energy is to tape the crystal to a small bottle of organic olive oil [100ml] – over time the crystal will infuse the oil with its properties and these are absorbed when you give yourself an abdominal massage with the oil.

If you don't like the feel of oil, do the same but with a bottle of spring water and a spray nozzle – and maybe add a drop of Lavender or Frankincense essential oil too. Give yourself a 'spritz' on your abdomen when you come out of the shower on damp skin.

My top favourites for digestion include:

AMBER – this is such an ancient, earthy 'crystal', it can absorb pain and negative energy, creating space for healing energies to flow. Especially good for Liver and Gallbladder.

FRANKINCENSE RESIN – OK, also not strictly a crystal but this resin is a fast and effective general 'balancer' – very effective in the oil mix or water spray mentioned above.

JASPER – is also known as the 'supreme nurturer' and supports the digestive system and helps balance emotional stress that may be aggravating your cantankerous gut.

MOONSTONE – always associated with the female organs and the feminine within, it is also excellent at calming the entire digestive tract.

OBSIDIAN – at the other end of the colour spectrum this dark stone is very useful in getting the system moving and removing blockages.

Remember – if you learn to energy test – the very best way of choosing your crystal is to test it.

Hold it against your abdomen and test –

- *Weak?* Then that crystal is not for you.
- *Strong?* Then it could be just what you need.

To make your test even more accurate:

Unzip [top to bottom direction] your central meridian [the line running up the centre of your torso from the pubic area to the bottom lip] – this will instantly 'weaken' you. Now hold the crystal against your abdomen and test:

- *Weak?* – this crystal is neutral, it doesn't actually strengthen you but neither does it weaken you

- *Strong?* – yes – success! <u>This is the crystal for you</u>, it has the ability to strengthen you from a weakened state.

Have fun with your crystal, clean it, clear it, connect with it and make it part of your life.

Colonic irrigation

Colonic Irrigation is an option you might like to consider for bowel health. I promise you it is not as bad you think it might be – quite relaxing, in fact almost pleasant! It is not necessarily something you will do every week for the rest of your life, but it can 'kick start' your intestine into a more normal function and certainly clean out any debris that may be lurking around potentially causing problems. Warm water[20] is pumped into the intestines and removed through a tube – nothing is seen, it is infinitely clean and comfortable.

If you are curious – visit You Tube there are a couple of very reassuring and instructional clips available.

GETTING A GOOD MOTION GOING

Another way of course of cleansing the gut is the Psyllium husk and bentolite clay mix mentioned earlier or some really good rustic rye bread with seeds or what works miracles for me is my favourite breakfast – guaranteed to promote good bowel movement:

- 1 kiwi fruit and a banana chopped up into little pieces and placed in a glass.
- 1 tablespoon of 'healthy' crunchy granola/muesli

---

[20] In the Indian tradition, warm oil is used instead of water in the belief that this is less 'aggressive' on the gut, strips it less and leaves it in a better condition.

- 1 tablespoon of unsweetened Greek yogurt or Quark
- Sprinkle with a few berries
- Sprinkle with a few finely chopped almonds
- Sprinkle with 2 tablespoons of split hemp seeds, linseeds and Chia
- You can add sesame or other seeds if you wish

A friend of mine who has always had problems with 'regularity' came to stay and in two days she was like clockwork – so thrilled was she that she rushed round to her local health store as soon as she got home and bought all the ingredients and now swears by her Maddie Brekkie.

Toilet training

FEET ON STOOL – anyone visiting my bathroom will see a little white plastic stool, only a few guess its use. Now you will all know: In a natural world the optimum position for a bowel movement is to squat, it opens up the area and puts us in the right 'angle'. Everything is open and gravity can lend a hand, making your 'motion' strain-free, more complete, quick and easy; as Nature intended.

It is not practical to squat on our Western loos so putting your feet on a stool [about 6" in height] creates a fair imitation.

Extra advice for the constipated

- What is a healthy bowel movement?
- Are you constipated without knowing it?

Just because you 'go' once a day, doesn't mean you are not constipated, you could be carrying around a few pounds of fermenting food that would be better eliminated. If not, it can begin to adhere and irritate the delicate lining of the lower intestine and cause no end of mischief.

Ideally, you should have an easy bowel movement when you get up and early afternoon and evening: it makes sense to work on the basis of: 'what goes in must come out'.

- Consistency should be medium – not too hard or too loose.
- Colour not too light, yellow or dark.
- Ideally it should sink not float.

Give yourself time, never ignore the urge to eliminate. We need to move waste through the system within 24 hours – not more than 36.

Constipation is normally caused by an unhealthy diet, lifestyle, dehydration, lack of exercise and of course, stress.

The more refined and white a diet the more there could be a problem. Turn to fresh fruit and veg and lots of water to flush through the intestines. I often grate carrots, broccoli, cabbage and pop in a few pieces of apple, kiwi fruit, figs and grapes: mix together with a light dressing of your choice to make a coleslaw with enough bulk to move things on and out.

Sprinkle flaxseeds [linseeds] or split hemp seeds on top of the coleslaw or on your morning cereal. I sometimes add a sprinkle of Lethicin over my food – it helps emulsify and digest fats.

MASSAGE

Coconut oil and Olive Oil can be your friends. Use whichever one you prefer externally for a deep abdominal massage [in a clockwise direction] and/or internally, take loads as a dressing on your salad. Buy the best quality you can afford or find.

Massage internally by deep breathing into the abdominal area, hold the breath there for a few seconds before breathing out slowly and pulling your navel in to touch your spine [okay, so this is physically impossible, but you get my meaning]. Repeat several times, eyes closed, connecting to your abdomen.

AFFIRMATIONS

While doing that you may like to make an affirmation to encourage 'movement'. For example...

> **I now release with ease all that needs to come out on both a physical and emotional level – all is well**

Each organ of the body has an emotional association: Large Intestine sits in Metal Element and that is related to 'letting go' – so what is it in your life that you need to now let go of?

Diarrhoea

First of all, start massaging the points on the outside of your thighs [mentioned earlier in the book] upwards from the knees to the hips. These are reflex points direct to the Large Intestine and the upward direction will encourage less of a *'downward movement'.*

Dehydration can be a problem with constant and aggressive Diarrhoea, so make sure you drink water.

Commonsense dictates that you should eat or drink nothing spicy or extreme in taste or texture. So bland food for a few days. Again, perhaps the best way of eating is to energy test everything before you ingest it – test before you ingest – to ensure you are not eating anything that will aggravate the problem.

Diarrhoea will normally clear itself in a couple of days if your immune system is strong. One way of helping your immune system is to strengthen your Spleen energy and you can do this by simply 'tracing' the Spleen pathway of energy.

Tracing is often dismissed as being too easy; but sometimes the simplest techniques are all that are needed to bring about a shift. Tracing is a fundamental tool of energy work. Your hands are like little electromagnetic pads and once aligned over the body; they connect with the body's energy and move it.

The rule is: move [i.e. trace] with the flow, the direction, of the meridian will strengthen in. Move backwards will weaken/ sedate it.

Sit down or stand and lean forward and place your fingertips onto the inside corner of each big toe – by 'inside' I mean the side next to the air, not the side next to the second toe.

Slowly bring your hands up over the top/side of the foot and then flatten your hands so your palms are against the body, either touching or slightly hovering. Trace straight up the inside of the legs. Fare out at the hips slightly. Come up the side of the ribcage to the armpit and then dip back down the ribcage to the bottom of the ribcage.

Smile as you do it and do it 3 times, maybe saying an affirmation of choice such as:

"my immune system is strong and my diarrhoea is disappearing fast as I return to health – all is well"

Follow with what I call a **MONKEY THUMP** which will:

- ✓ Lift your energy level
- ✓ Balance your blood chemistry and hormones
- ✓ Strengthen your immune system and remove toxins thus helping bring an end to the diarrhoea
- ✓ Synchronise your body's rhythms
- ✓ Help you not only metabolise food more efficiently but also the inevitable challenges that life presents!

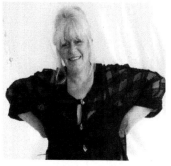

- • Clench your fists and with the circle formed with the thumb and index finger,
- • Thump underneath your armpit [à la monkey!]
- • Your hands will be over the area of the side of your bra [Spleen 21].
- • Tap over these meridian points for a few seconds, don't hold your breath!

I love these points, however Donna Eden [Eden Energy Medicine] loves the Spleen Neurolymphatic points even more. So, a cunning way to stimulate them both is: after tapping the meridian points for a few seconds, keep tapping, change your hand position from a clenched fist to a triad [thumb and first two fingers straight and together] and tap around the ribs, under the breasts onto the NLRPs – ouch! Probably it hurts, but then you know you need it!

You can end with a:

TRIPLE WARMER/SPLEEN CUDDLE

Wrap your right hand around your left rib cage, over the spleen, forearm under the breasts. Left hand wraps around the top of the right arm [over TW points]. Hug yourself in this way and swing gently from side to side.

Summary

I hope there is something in this little book that you feel will be useful to you or that you can pass on to a friend or family member. To summarise ways you can help your digestion; you can consider:

- Reducing your **stress** and anxiety, giving your digestion a chance to return to harmony
- Formulating a **diet** that suits your own personal body chemistry – maybe consider for a few weeks the 'test before you ingest' way of eating. Or certainly identifying, through testing or observation, those foods that your digestion struggles with, and avoiding them

- Drinking plenty of **water** to benefit the entire tract and lessen the chances of constipation or dehydration
- Talk to your local nutritional adviser regarding suitable **supplements**, or, if you are confident with your self testing; test to see which strengthen you and are therefore right for you at the moment
- Introduce **Flower essences** and **essential oils** into your life
- Try a simple **Chakra** Balance over the abdominal area
- Trace your **energy** pathways
- Hold the powerful **source points** on the wrists and ankles to hyperlink some energy to the organs
- Hold/massage the digestive '**system point**'
- **Massage** the abdomen, the points on the inside and outside of your thighs
- Clear the Houston and Illeocecal **valves** in the shower
- **Stretch,** exercise and **walk**
- Consider **crystals**
- **Colonic** irrigation, use a stool in the bathroom [oops, excuse the pun]
- Dry **skin brushing**
- Strengthen your **Spleen energy** and therefore immunity
- Make use of simple **affirmations** while doing any of the above

Madison 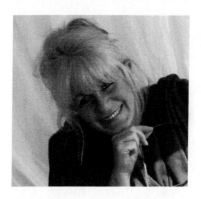 King

Writer & Teacher of Energy Medicine

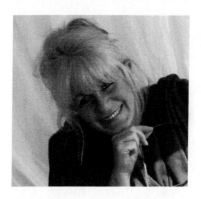

Madison's Medicine is a unique fusion of energy and body work, flower essences, lifestyle advice and commonsense – providing essential, everyday, practical tools for a healthier and happier you.

Many moons ago Madison was involved in the heart of London advertising, becoming a successful international board director. However, she realised, after a few ambition fuelled years, that she wanted her life to take a different direction and shocked everyone by giving up the BMW, Armani suits and Gucci briefcase, becoming a student again.

She trained in massage, sports massage, aromatherapy, Indian head massage, reflexology, trager, nutrition, flower essences, crystals, radionics... A true workshop groupie, she filled a wall with qualifications but could not find what she had been seeking; she couldn't even really define it... until, through divine synchronicity, she met Donna Eden in London through a mutual friend. Within no time at all she was in Ashland in Donna's backyard with about four other students, eagerly learning about energy – this was more than two decades ago, so no information highway was available in those days and ever the thirsty student she drank in everything she could on these visits, rushing back to London to experiment on her long suffering clients!

Over the years she crossed the ocean many times learning from Donna and also John Thie [Touch for Health].

She then began to teach Donna's work in the UK, USA, Gozo, Malta, Italy, Egypt and many other locations around the world, she has appeared on national UK television, radio and press promoting EEM. She has lectured at Westminster and Oxford universities and at the key Mind Body Spirit Festivals in London and Wales.

In 2006 she gave up a thriving practice in Central London and now divides her time between the Isle of Wight and the Andalucían town of Nerja in Southern Spain.

Just entering her 7th decade, she has set up and is running Donna Eden's training in Europe – based just outside London in Dorking... a long way from those days in Donna's back yard!

Her focus is on promoting Eden Energy Medicine in Europe and also writing and teaching her own very down to earth version: Madison's Medicine; which based on EEM also weaves in many other natural health threads, giving people simple yet powerful tools to enhance their quality of life on every single level.

As we enter unprecedented waters on this planet, it can be empowering to know that there is always something YOU can do to improve any situation, challenge or trauma that life throws into your path.

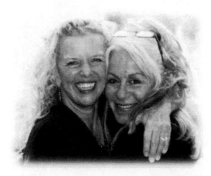

"Madison is an extraordinary woman and healer. She carries an essence of the highest quality and caring, of camaraderie of spirit, wisdom, compassion and depth of understanding of the healing realms. To train with her is something you will never regret"

Donna Eden – Eden Energy Medicine

www.madisonking.com
Facebook: Madison's Medicine
www.midlifegoddess.ning.com
madisonking@hotmail.com

My special thanks to Donna Eden.[21]

Without her friendship and generous, unselfish sharing of her vast knowledge, I would not be who I am today and you would not be reading this book.

I would also like to thank Anna Maria for her wonderful drawings that I hope you agree bring a clarity, lightness and warmth to the text. From her eyrie in Italy the images coming buzzing over to me with great enthusiasm and fun.

This is meant as a fun, useful guide to energy medicine and the digestive system, if it whets your appetite [another pun] for more information, visit my site: www.midlifegoddess.ning.com for up-to-date details on workshops, classes, weekly 'bite size', monthly online study groups, other books in the Essential Series, pdf downloads and my DVD or, if you prefer,

Facebook: Madison's Medicine for info, clips etc.,

Donna Eden's site. I strongly recommend her book

Energy Medicine

www.innersource.net

You Tube for some great clips – just tap in my name. Email me directly on madisonking@hotmail.com – I try and answer every email personally.

[21] www.innersource.net

Other books in the Essential Series include:

1. *Everyday Energy*

2. *Coping with Candida*

3. *Stiff Joints*

4. *MONEY* ... it's not a 4-lettered word. Connecting to your Universal Piggy Bank

And coming shortly, which is a companion to You've Got Guts: a book on Liver and Gallbladder [title not yet confirmed].

We aim to build this series to 30+ titles so join Madison's Midlife Goddess site or Facebook page for regular updates as the books become available.